Cambridge Elements ☰

Elements in Molecular Oncology
edited by
Edward P. Gelmann
University of Arizona

THERAPEUTIC TARGETING
OF RAS MUTANT CANCERS

Edward C. Stites
Salk Institute for Biological Studies

Kendra Paskvan
Pacific Northwest University for Health Sciences

Shumei Kato
University of California San Diego

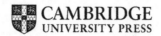
CAMBRIDGE
UNIVERSITY PRESS

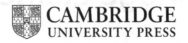

CAMBRIDGE
UNIVERSITY PRESS

Shaftesbury Road, Cambridge CB2 8EA, United Kingdom

One Liberty Plaza, 20th Floor, New York, NY 10006, USA

477 Williamstown Road, Port Melbourne, VIC 3207, Australia

314–321, 3rd Floor, Plot 3, Splendor Forum, Jasola District Centre,
New Delhi – 110025, India

103 Penang Road, #05–06/07, Visioncrest Commercial, Singapore 238467

Cambridge University Press is part of Cambridge University Press & Assessment,
a department of the University of Cambridge.

We share the University's mission to contribute to society through the pursuit of
education, learning and research at the highest international levels of excellence.

www.cambridge.org
Information on this title: www.cambridge.org/9781009073646

DOI: 10.1017/9781009064828

First published 2022

A catalogue record for this publication is available from the British Library.

ISBN 978-1-009-07364-6 Paperback
ISSN 2634-7490 (online)
ISSN 2634-7482 (print)

Therapeutic Targeting of RAS Mutant Cancers

Elements in Molecular Oncology

DOI: 10.1017/9781009064828
First published online: August 2022

Edward C. Stites
Salk Institute for Biological Studies

Kendra Paskvan
Pacific Northwest University for Health Sciences

Shumei Kato
University of California San Diego

Author for correspondence: Edward C. Stites, estites@salk.edu

Abstract: The KRAS oncogene is believed to be the most common single nucleotide variant oncogene in human cancer. Historically, efforts to target KRAS and the other RAS GTPases have struggled. More recently, efforts have focused on identifying and exploiting features unique to specific oncogenic mutations. This has led to the first FDA approval for a RAS targeted therapy. This new agent is a covalent inhibitor that reacts with the cysteine residue created by a codon 12 glycine to cysteine (G12C) mutation within KRAS. Mutant-specific strategies may also exist for other KRAS single nucleotide variants, and recent studies provide examples and mechanisms.

Keywords: KRAS, covalent inhibitor, targeted therapy, personalized medicine, G12C

ISBNs: 9781009073646 (PB), 9781009064828 (OC)
ISSNs: 2634-7490 (online), 2634-7482 (print)

Contents

1 Introduction

The 2021 FDA approval of Lumakras (sotorasib) [1] for lung cancer patients with the KRAS G12C mutation represents a major milestone in cancer therapeutics. This achievement, which comes approximately 40 years from the publication describing RAS as the first human oncogene to be discovered [2], may very well be the first of many more RAS-directed therapeutics to be approved for clinical use this upcoming decade.

The RAS GTPases (KRAS, NRAS, and HRAS) play major roles in human cancer (Figure 1). According to the National Cancer Institute (NCI) RAS Initiative, more than 30 percent of human cancers are driven by a mutation in one of these three RAS genes [3]. *KRAS* is the most commonly mutated of the three RAS genes. *KRAS* mutations can be detected in nearly all pancreatic adenocarcinomas [4, 5] and approximately 30 to 40 percent of lung adenocarcinomas and colorectal adenocarcinomas [6, 7]. *NRAS* mutations are observed in approximately 20 percent of malignant melanomas [8], and *HRAS* mutations are observed in head and neck cancers [9] as well as in bladder cancers [10] (Figure 2). These examples highlight some of the cancers in which the RAS genes are most commonly mutated; however, mutations to these genes are encountered to a lesser extent in a much wider variety of cancers.

RAS mutations have been linked to several important cancer phenotypes (Figure 3). Perhaps most importantly, RAS mutations are typically capable of conferring the "self-sufficiency in growth signals" cancer hallmark [11, 12]. This is critical for the dysregulated, elevated proliferation common to malignant tumors. Additionally, RAS mutations have been linked to metabolic phenotypes that appear critical to cancer [13–15] and to increased pro-survival signaling [16, 17].

2 RAS Biology

Several aspects of RAS targeting, including KRAS G12C targeting, are best understood after a review of the fundamental aspects of RAS biochemistry (Figure 4). To begin with, RAS has a nucleotide-binding pocket that can bind the guanosine nucleotides GTP and GDP. RAS proteins adopt different structural conformations on the basis of whether GTP or GDP is bound [18]. Downstream effector proteins bind specifically to the GTP-bound form of RAS (whether wild-type or mutant). The RAS-effector complex may be further modulated (such as by phosphorylation of the bound effector protein) as part of the transmission of RAS-GTP-dependent signals downstream from RAS through the effector [19]. RAS downstream effectors include the RAF kinases (BRAF, CRAF, and ARAF) as well as the phosphoinositide 3-kinases (*3*).

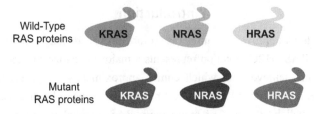

Figure 1 The RAS proteins.

The three RAS GTPases most associated with cancer are KRAS, NRAS, and HRAS. The wild-type RAS are cell signaling proteins that carry a variety of signals, including those for cellular proliferation. Mutant forms of RAS proteins are commonly found in cancer and are critical drivers of the cancer phenotype.

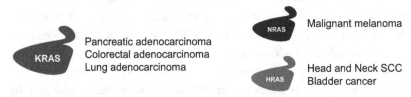

Figure 2 Mutant RAS proteins are common in many forms of cancer.

Mutant KRAS is found in a high proportion of pancreatic, colorectal, and lung adeno-carcinoma patients. Mutant NRAS is common in malignant melanoma. Mutant HRAS is commonly observed in head and neck squamous cell carcinoma and bladder carcinoma.

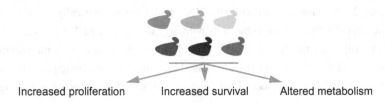

Figure 3 Mutant RAS phenotypes.

Mutant RAS proteins are associated with several important cancer phenotypes. These mutants are well-established drivers of increased cellular proliferation. RAS mutants have also been implicated with increased cellular survival signals and metabolic alter-ations that support increased cancer cell proliferation.

The level of GTP-RAS is therefore a critical variable that governs cellular phenotypes. The cellular level of GTP-RAS and GDP-RAS reflects a dynamic equilibrium between several processes. RAS itself is a GTPase, as it can catalyze the hydrolysis of GTP to GDP [20]. This reaction is generally slow, and GAP proteins (GTPase Activating Proteins) can expedite GTP hydrolysis [21]. RAS GTPases bind to guanosine nucleotides with very high affinity, and spontaneous dissociation of GTP and GDP by a free RAS protein is very slow [20]. GEF proteins (Guanine Nucleotide Exchange Factors) reduce the affinity

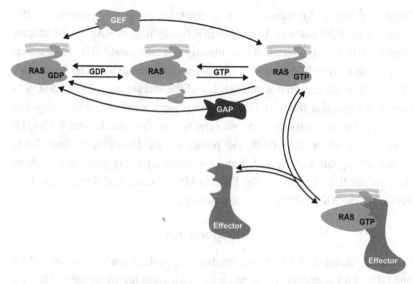

Figure 4 The RAS nucleotide exchange cycle.
Cellular levels of GDP-bound RAS (the inactive form of RAS) and GTP-bound RAS (the active form of RAS) are controlled by a variety of biochemical processes. RAS GEFs promote nucleotide dissociation and exchange, and tend to promote net conversion to GTP-bound RAS due to the cellular excess of GTP over GDP. Spontaneous nucleotide dissociation without a GEF can also occur at much slower rates for wild-type RAS. Some oncogenic RAS mutants, however, have significantly elevated spontaneous nucleotide dissociation (and activation). RAS-GTP may be converted to RAS-GDP directly through the GTPase activity of RAS. RAS-GAPs, however, are much stronger promoters of RAS-GTP-to-RAS-GDP conversion. Most oncogenic RAS proteins are completely to strongly resistant to the activity of GAP proteins. RAS effector proteins specifically bind to RAS-GTP.

of RAS for its nucleotides and increase the dissociation rate for nucleotides [22]. As there is an approximately 10:1 excess of GTP to GDP in the cell [23], nucleotide exchange tends to result in the conversion of GDP-bound RAS for GTP-bound RAS. Effector proteins also contribute to the dynamic equilibrium, as effectors, GAPs, and GEFs bind to RAS in an overlapping region that includes the nucleotide binding pocket. Thus, these reactions are competitive, and the binding of RAS-GTP to a GAP, GEF, or effector can effectively prevent the simultaneous binding of another RAS binding partner.

As mentioned earlier, the RAS GTPases are signaling proteins and they are critical to the transmission of signals from surface receptors. One significant surface receptor that signals through RAS is the Epidermal Growth Factor Receptor (EGFR). The activation of EGFR by one of its ligands leads to activation of the EGFR kinase domain, trans-autophosphorylation of the EGFR dimer [24], and the recruitment of SH2 and PTB domain containing "reader" proteins that transmit signals downstream to many pathways [25], including the RAS pathway. Critical to EGFR activation of RAS are the adapter proteins SHC1 [26], which can bind directly to EGFR, and GRB2 [27], which can bind directly to EGFR as well as to phosphorylated SHC1. The RAS GEFs SOS1 and SOS2 can bind with GRB2, and the recruitment of GRB2/SOS is critical for bringing the SOS GEFs to the plasma membrane where they can activate RAS. By "activate RAS" we refer to a net increase in total RAS-GTP from a state where RAS-GDP had predominated. Downstream from RAS, RAS-GTP signals may spread through distinct signaling pathways, such as through the RAF kinases to the ERK/MAPK cascade and through the PI3-kinases to the AKT/mTOR survival pathway.

3 Oncogenic RAS

Within an oncogenic RAS mutant, the dynamic equilibrium between GTP-RAS and GDP-RAS is strongly perturbed such that a much higher fraction of RAS is bound to GTP (Figure 5). The term "constitutively active" is commonly used to describe this state of the dynamic equilibrium where GTP-bound levels are relatively high. Over the years, the term "constitutively active" has commonly been misconstrued to mean that the individual RAS proteins are each "locked" into a GTP-bound state. However, cellular measurements of mutant RAS-GTP and GDP suggest that oncogenic RAS is not all RAS-GTP bound [28, 29]. This point is important to consider for KRAS G12C inhibitors, which will be discussed in Section 8 of this Element.

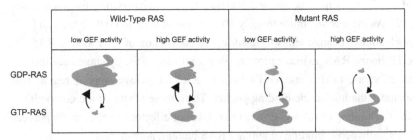

The dynamic equilibrium between GDP- and GTP-bound RAS is influenced by whether the RAS protein is wild-type or mutant, and by levels of cellular GEF activity

Figure 5 The RAS dynamic equilibrium in wild-type and mutant RAS. Levels of GDP- and GTP-bound wild-type RAS are dynamically controlled, predominantly by GEF and GAP activities. Wild-type RAS is predominantly GDP bound unless cellular GEF activity is elevated. Mutant RAS is predominantly GTP bound regardless of cellular GEF activity. Cellular GEF activity, though, may further increase cellular RAS-GTP levels.

There are many different RAS single nucleotide variants that may be observed in human cancer [20, 30]. Most of the oncogenic RAS alleles are constitutively active due to the presence of a point mutation that prevents RAS-GAPs from being able to promote the GTP-to-GDP conversion. This is usually thought of as an absolute elimination of GAP activity, although some RAS mutants may still display a very low level of sensitivity to GAP inactivation [31–33]. As GAP-mediated conversion of RAS-GTP to RAS-GDP is the dominant mechanism of wild-type (WT) RAS inactivation, an oncogenic RAS mutant's loss of sensitivity to GAP-mediated inactivation strongly shifts the dynamic equilibrium toward increased levels of GTP-bound RAS.

Despite an insensitivity to GAP-mediated GTP-to-GDP conversion, oncogenic RAS-GTP can still be converted to RAS-GDP through intrinsic GTPase activity (which is also typically partially impaired in oncogenic mutants). Additionally, nucleotide exchange should result in loading of oncogenic RAS with GDP rather than GTP approximately 10 percent of the time. These mechanisms of conversion of oncogenic RAS-GTP to oncogenic RAS-GDP are important to note because the KRAS G12C inhibitors that are currently in clinical trial bind specifically to the GDP-bound form of mutant RAS. Thus, mechanisms that result in conversion of GTP-mutant RAS to GDP-mutant RAS are of more than academic interest.

4 RAS Targeting

Oncogenic RAS has long been seen as a potentially valuable therapeutic target. That RAS could be a valuable target is supported by a range of data that suggest RAS cancers retain a dependency on the presence of the RAS mutation for ongoing survival [34, 35]. This ongoing dependence on the presence of the oncogenic mutation is known as "oncogene addiction," and it provides a philosophical basis for many targeted therapies [36].

Targeting RAS directly at the nucleotide-binding pocket may seem like a valuable strategy that would be analogous to the targeting of protein kinases with small molecules that bind the ATP binding pocket. However, the RAS GTPases bind GTP and GDP with picomolar affinity, while kinases tend to bind ATP with millimolar affinity [3]. Thus, the million- to billionfold difference in affinity presents a very large obstacle for the development of RAS nucleotide-binding pocket inhibitors. Additionally, the high cellular levels of GTP and GDP [23] would further make it exceptionally hard for a small molecule to outcompete GTP and GDP to bind to an accessible pocket.

The pharmaceutical industry put a tremendous amount of effort into developing small molecules that prevent the proper membrane localization of RAS.

RAS is post-translationally modified on its C-terminus, where it may be farnesylated [37]. The farnesyl transferase inhibitors (FTIs) attracted the most attention in this category. Preclinical studies in mouse models suggested that FTI could be useful [38], although clinical trial results were much less promising [37]. One possible reason for the disappointing clinical trial studies could be off-target toxicity, as many proteins other than RAS are farnesylated. Additionally, studies suggested that KRAS and NRAS could obtain proper membrane localization through alternative post-translational lipid modification pathways [39, 40]. Surprisingly, although the field considered FTI to only potentially be useful for HRAS mutant cancers due to the alternative modification pathways for KRAS and NRAS, there does not seem to have been a significant effort to adapt FTI to HRAS mutant cancers at that time. Over the past decade, however, it seems that interest in considering FTI for HRAS mutant cancers has increased [41]. For example, Ho and colleagues recently evaluated tipifarnib (an FTI) for recurrent and metastatic head and neck squamous cell carcinoma with HRAS mutation, and they observed a 55 percent response rate ($N = 20$ evaluable patients) [42]. This renewed interest may reflect a trend where personalized cancer medicine is willing to consider smaller and smaller molecularly defined subsets of cancer as viable patient populations for targeting.

5 Downstream Targeting

Due to the challenges of targeting RAS directly, there has been much interest in targeting the signals that propagate from RAS through other proteins. The successful development of kinase inhibitors made kinases an appealing target, and the RAF and PI3 K proteins that are RAS effector proteins are kinases. At this time, however, no RAF or PI3 K inhibitor that has advanced to clinical trials has proven useful for RAS mutant cancers [30]. Consideration of inhibitors in the RAF/MEK/ERK pathway illuminates some of the complexity that comes with targeting downstream from RAS.

Although several RAF kinase inhibitors have been developed, they do not appear useful as a single agent against RAS mutant cancers. Indeed, RAF kinase inhibitors can actually increase the total level of oncogenic RAS signal through a process commonly referred to as "paradoxical activation" [43, 44]. For example, BRAF mutant melanoma patients treated with a BRAF inhibitor commonly develop cutaneous squamous cell carcinomas, and these squamous cell carcinomas commonly have an HRAS mutation whose signal is further potentiated (thereby driving increased proliferation) by the BRAF inhibitor [45]. Paradoxical activation is not completely understood, but it involves the

RAF-inhibitor-stabilizing RAF dimers that are critical for transmitting RAS signals. Ongoing work in BRAF inhibitor development aims to develop improved RAF inhibitors that may be less prone to paradoxical activation [46]. It is possible that BRAF inhibitors will someday be developed that prove useful for RAS mutant cancer patients.

MEK inhibitors would also be anticipated to be useful in RAS mutant cancers and should not display RAF paradoxical activation. In practice, however, MEK inhibitors have not proven useful in RAS mutant cancer [47, 48]. Intriguingly, MEK inhibitors recently demonstrated benefit in clinical trials for patients with neurofibromatosis [49]. Neurofibromatosis is a genetic disease that is caused by a germline mutation in the gene *NF1* that codes for the RAS-GAP neurofibromin. Increased levels of wild-type RAS-GTP result from the decrease in functional neurofibromin proteins that follows from such mutations, and increased RAS-GTP is believed to be critical to the development of the pleiotropic neurofibromatosis phenotypes. That MEK inhibitors offered benefit suggests that these MEK inhibitors can offer clinical benefit via inhibiting pathological RAS signals, and some personalized medicine clinical trials that use MEK inhibitors "off label" have reported overall positive trends [50, 51]. However, clinical trials that focus on the treatment of RAS mutant cancers with a MEK inhibitor have found little to no benefit [47, 52, 53]. One of the challenges with MEK inhibition could be co-genomic alteration that is associated with RAS alterations. We have previously reported that 95 percent of cancers with RAS mutations also harbor co-alterations (median of 3). The most common co-alterations that may explain limited efficacy with MEK inhibitors alone were found in the PI3 K pathway (31%), in cell cycle pathways (31%), in tyrosine kinases (22%), and in BRCA-associated genes (13%) [54]. Hence, targeting co-genomic alterations along with MEK inhibition may be necessary for RAS-altered cancers [55, 56].

6 Upstream Targeting

The presence of a RAS mutation is widely believed to indicate resistance to EGFR inhibitors in both colorectal and lung cancers [57, 58]. However, erlotinib was FDA approved in pancreatic adenocarcinoma on the basis of a response duration of less than two weeks [59]. As KRAS mutations are almost universally present in pancreas cancer [4, 5], even a partial benefit is notable. More intriguingly, analyses of phase III clinical trials suggest that EGFR inhibitor cetuximab may offer benefit in KRAS G13D mutant colorectal cancer [60, 61], a topic that will be further addressed in Section 11 of this Element.

Perhaps less controversial will be the utilization of inhibitors with targets between the receptor tyrosine kinases and RAS. Inhibitors to SHP2 (*PTPN11*) and SOS1/2 fit this description. SOS1/2 are GEF proteins, and their activity on RAS is clear: they promote nucleotide exchange, and targeting SOS1/2 could potentially tip the dynamic equilibrium toward a state with less total RAS-GTP. Several groups have pursued SOS inhibitors to different extents [62–64], and one SOS inhibitor (BI 1701963, Boehringer Ingelheim) has advanced to clinical trial. SHP2 inhibitors are also in clinical trial, and these inhibitors are believed to result in reduced signaling within the RAS pathway. The mechanism by which the phosphatase SHP2 contributes to RAS pathway activation is not fully understood, but it appears that SHP2 phosphatase activity can counteract phosphorylation events that drive processes that negatively regulate RAS signals [65]. Thus, SHP2 activity promotes RAS pathway signaling, and SHP2 inhibition reduces RAS pathway signaling. Whether SHP2 inhibition offers benefit in RAS mutant cancers remains to be determined.

7 Targeting Specific RAS Mutants

The most commonly encountered oncogenic RAS alleles occur at codons 12, 13, or 61 [30]. Different specific amino acid substitution mutations may be observed at each of these hot spots. For example, G12D, G12V, and G12C mutations are the most common oncogenic variants observed at codon 12. Codon 13 is, coincidentally, also normally a glycine ("G"), and it is most commonly mutated to an aspartic acid ("D") in human cancer.

Biophysically, the major hot-spot oncogenic RAS mutants are impaired at GAP inactivation, and this defect accounts for the majority of their net shift to a GTP-bound state [66]. However, each of the amino acid substitutions introduces a slightly different collection of atoms into the RAS three-dimensional structure and also introduces different variations in the electrostatics of the region. Biophysically, the different substitution mutations also alter the chemical kinetics of all the other biochemical reactions that relate to RAS signaling, and the magnitude of the variations can vary between substituting mutations [20, 67]. Many of the exciting advances in RAS targeting come from a renewed interest in studying and exploiting these differences.

8 KRAS G12C Targeting

The major breakthrough that catalyzed a renewed interest in RAS therapeutics involved the development of covalent inhibitors that target the KRAS G12C mutation (Figure 6). This is the most common KRAS mutation in lung cancer [68]. This mutation is, however, uncommon in pancreatic cancer [4, 5] and in

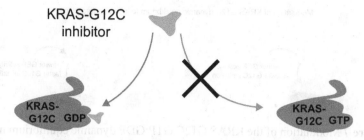

Figure 6 Small molecular targeting of KRAS G12C.
Small molecule inhibitors that specifically react with KRAS G12C and covalently bond with the cysteine residue at codon 12 have been described to exclusively to strongly favor the GDP-bound form of KRAS G12C.

colorectal cancer [7]. The field of RAS cancer therapeutics changed dramatically with the development and description of small molecules that specifically covalently react with the cysteine residue of KRAS G12C [69]. This demonstrated the value of this approach to the broader scientific and medical communities. In parallel and in follow-up studies, a variety of pharmaceutical and biotech companies have also advanced KRAS G12C inhibitor programs [1, 70–72].

Importantly, this original study [69] also found that, after covalently reacting with the codon 12 cysteine, the small molecule inhibitor also nestled into a new, previously unknown pocket on the surface of RAS [69]. Thus, in addition to identifying a new strategy for targeting RAS, this work also suggested that there may be other unknown opportunities to target RAS.

One important consideration as these inhibitors move into the clinic is whether the benefit of the inhibitor can be increased by the addition of another targeted therapy. Notably, and perhaps surprisingly, EGFR inhibitors have been suggested to be a promising agent for combination with G12C inhibitors. This is supported by a variety of preclinical in vivo and in vitro studies [1, 70, 71, 73–78]. One mechanism that has been proposed to explain why EGFR inhibitors increase the benefit of G12C inhibitors is that the G12C inhibitors bind specifically to the inactive, GDP-bound form of KRAS G12C. This may at first be superficially surprising because it is common to think of oncogenic RAS as constitutively active and as GTP bound [73, 79]. However, a dynamic equilibrium exists, and oncogenic RAS may be found in both GDP- and GTP-bound forms, although the net balance within oncogenic RAS mutants tends to overwhelmingly favor the GTP-bound state (Figure 7). One reason that EGFR inhibition has been promoted to increase the effects of KRAS G12C inhibitors is that it may help suppress the conversion of GDP-bound KRAS G12C to GTP-bound KRAS G12C [73]. As EGFR activation can lead to RAS activation, and as EGFR activation plays an important role in

Modulation of KRAS G12C dynamic equilibrium to increase targeting

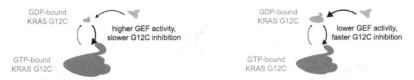

Figure 7 Modulation of the KRAS G12C GTP:GDP dynamic equilibrium may improve G12C targeting.

Many preclinical studies have found that EGFR inhibitors potentiate the ability of G12C inhibitors to bind to KRAS G12C. This is believed to in part follow from EGFR inhibition leading to reduced GEF activity, in turn shifting the dynamic equilibrium of KRAS G12C to a state with increased GDP-bound KRAS G12C that can then be targeted by the G12C inhibitor.

non–small-cell lung cancer, it seems reasonable to consider that there is some basal signaling from EGFR to RAS that may be partially suppressed with an EGFR inhibitor.

Another mechanism that has been argued to contribute to the value of EGFR inhibitors in combination with KRAS G12C inhibitors involves negative feedback [76]. Multiple negative feedback processes exist in the cell that combat aberrant activation of the RAS pathway. Thus, a KRAS G12C cancer cell typically has an elevated RAS pathway signal that promotes cellular proliferation despite stronger-than-normal inhibition of the EGFR/RAS/ERK pathway through activated negative feedback processes. Once RAS is inhibited, there is typically a very strong, initial, transient suppression, as the oncogene has been targeted and the strong negative feedback operates unopposed. The profound suppression of signal eliminates the ongoing induction of signals that promote negative feedback, and the negative feedback processes are reduced. The cell then "reactivates" to a new level that is typically assumed to be less than what was experienced before treatment was initiated, but that will be above the low level of signal that was caused by initial targeting. If this new level of reactivation (where the oncogene may only be partially inhibited, and where less negative feedback is present) is sufficient to drive proliferation, the treatment will not be fully effective. Targeting EGFR is believed to help block the reactivation of the EGFR/RAS/ERK pathway [80, 81]. This has perhaps best been described in *BRAF* mutant colorectal cancers, where a treatment regimen that combines an EGFR inhibitor along with a BRAF and MEK inhibitor has proven useful in phase three clinical trials, and where the believed mechanism is the blocking of feedback reactivation [53].

As KRAS G12C inhibitors are newly FDA approved and much research is ongoing, it is possible that additional benefits of the combination of G12C inhibitors with EGFR inhibitors will be identified. It is also likely that other targets for combination therapy will be identified. For example, newly developed agents against SHP2 appear to offer benefit when combined with KRAS G12C inhibitors, potentially because they can broadly counteract RTK activation of RAS [76].

Another major issue of clinical importance will be how resistance develops within KRAS G12C mutant tumors that are treated with a KRAS G12C inhibitor. Resistance against anticancer agents is a major obstacle that can limit the duration of benefit from pharmacologics. Reports of acquired clinical resistance to G12C inhibitors are just beginning to emerge [82]. Early work studying clinical resistance within a single clinical trial patient observed the outgrowth of cancerous cells that harbored KRAS, NRAS, BRAF, and MAP2K1 (coding for MEK1) mutations [83]. The acquisition of new mutations that confer the RAS activation phenotype and are insensitive to the drug being used mirrors clinical resistance with other targeted therapies, and the acquisition of a new mutant within the same gene (a Y96D mutation in cis with G12C) that reduces the ability of the targeted therapy to engage.

9 Direct Targeting of Other RAS Proteins

The development of KRAS G12C inhibitors may have opened a Pandora's box for the consideration of each RAS mutation as a distinct entity, in contrast to the goal of finding a single strategy that targets most RAS mutants. One could envision novel strategies to target oncogenic RAS at the DNA, RNA, or peptide level on the basis of the unique oncogenic sequences. In principle, such approaches could be developed for each oncogenic RAS mutant. Multiple vaccine strategies have been and are being pursued along these lines. Notably, Moderna, the company that successfully introduced the mRNA COVID-19 vaccine, has an oncogenic RAS mRNA vaccine in clinical trial [84].

The aforementioned unique physicochemical aspects of each amino acid substitution and its interactions with structurally nearby residues may create uniquely reactive opportunities for small molecule targeting. Small molecules that target other specific KRAS mutations are reportedly in development. For example, Mirati Therapeutics, one of the first companies to advance a KRAS G12C inhibitor into clinical trial [71], is developing a first-in-class inhibitor for targeting KRAS G12D. This compound, which they refer to as MRTX1133, is described as having low nanomolar potency, to be selective for the KRAS G12D mutant but not KRAS WT tumors, and to bind both active and inactive forms of

KRAS G12D. Other RAS mutant-specific drug development programs are reportedly underway in multiple companies, but detailed information on strategies is not being publicly disclosed.

The development of novel small molecules, biologics, vaccines, and immunotherapies that target RAS will be an exciting story to monitor over the upcoming decade. In parallel, recently published work on mutant-specific signaling differences with clinical target implications may provide a preview of what is to come.

10 KRAS G12R Pancreatic Cancer

Recent studies suggest that KRAS G12R cancers may have unique, targetable vulnerabilities [85]. KRAS G12R is common in pancreatic cancer, but is much less common in other forms of cancer that frequently harbor a KRAS mutation. Experimental studies that compared pancreatic cancer cells with the KRAS G12R mutation against pancreatic cancer cells with other KRAS mutations observed that the KRAS mutant-dependent micropinocytosis commonly observed in pancreatic cancer cells that harbor a KRAS G12D or KRAS G12V mutation [14] was not observed in KRAS G12R mutant pancreatic cancer cells [85].

Structurally, KRAS G12R was found to have a disrupted structure for its GTP-bound state relative to the form of other oncogenic KRAS alleles bound to GTP. This structural difference was observed to reduce nucleotide exchange by SOS1 and to reduce binding to PI3 Kα, and the reduction in PI3 Kα binding was the attributed cause of impaired micropinocytosis promotion by KRAS G12R relative to the other KRAS mutations.

The authors of this study [85] also observed that KRAS G12R pancreatic cancer cell lines, organoids, and xenografts were relatively more sensitive to the MEK inhibitor selumetinib than were cancer cell lines, organoids, and xenografts that harbored other KRAS mutations. The authors also noted screens that suggested other possible mutant-specific combinations that should be further studied and validated for benefit to KRAS G12R mutant pancreatic adenocarcinoma patients. Overall, this study highlights that, in addition to the introduction of mutant-specific, chemically reactive residues (like G12C), mutations can also disrupt protein–protein interactions and reaction kinetics and thereby alter relative sensitivity to anticancer therapeutics.

11 KRAS G13D Colorectal Cancer

Another RAS mutation that has evidence for being clinically actionable is KRAS G13D, found most commonly in colorectal cancers. It has been common practice to consider all codon 12, 13, and 61 KRAS and NRAS mutations biomarkers for resistance to EGFR inhibition [86]. This is on the basis of pooling all mutant-positive patients into a cohort and comparing their overall response to treatment with the pool of all RAS wild-type patients [57]. Although the different oncogenic RAS mutants are constitutively active, the mutant-to-mutant specific differences in biochemical and biophysical properties that may result in biological differences in signaling suggest that such groupings must be considered carefully.

Two retrospective analyses of the Phase III clinical trials that considered different, specific, mutant alleles suggested that patients with the KRAS G13D mutation were sensitive to treatment with the EGFR inhibitor cetuximab [60, 61]. However, this observation was controversial [87], and other retrospective analyses of other trials suggested no benefit from EGFR inhibition in KRAS G13D colorectal cancers [88]. What has become less controversial is that KRAS G13D has several notable biochemical differences from the other common hot-spot KRAS mutations. Firstly, KRAS G13D has been noted to have a reduced affinity for GTP and GDP, and non–GEF-mediated nucleotide exchange occurs at a much higher rate for KRAS G13D [20]. Additionally, although KRAS G13D is impaired at GAP-mediated GTP hydrolysis, like other oncogenic mutants, the extent of the reduction is less absolute [31–33]. Additionally, the binding affinity between KRAS G13D and the RAS-GAP neurofibromin appears to be significantly reduced [89, 90].

Two prospective, randomized control, Phase II clinical trials were performed to evaluate the treatment of colorectal cancer patients with cetuximab [91, 92]. However, both trials compared cetuximab treatment to cetuximab and irinotecan, so only irinotecan varied between groups. Although the observations of both studies were similar, one group concluded that cetuximab likely offered a benefit and the other reported that cetuximab did not likely offer a benefit. A prospective trial comparing a treatment regimen that includes cetuximab (or another EGFR inhibitor) with the same treatment regimen absent the EGFR inhibitor has not been performed, so the clinical benefit of EGFR inhibition in colorectal cancer patients remains unclear.

Two recent studies have investigated a mechanism for why KRAS G13D cancers may respond to EGFR-directed treatment [32, 33, 90]. These studies may lead to a reconsideration of cetuximab (or panitumumab) as an option for KRAS G13D colorectal cancer treatment. The first study used a mathematical model of the processes that regulate the RAS nucleotide binding dynamic equilibrium to investigate the different, common, KRAS mutations and their response to EGFR inhibition [90]. Surprisingly, the mathematical model suggested that the available biochemical data on biochemical reactions was sufficient to provide a mechanistic explanation for why KRAS G13D cancers may be relatively more sensitive to EGFR inhibition. As the clinical trial evidence had been dismissed by the community in part due to the assumption that all constitutively active RAS mutants would behave similarly, this was a notable computational finding. Similarly, the fact that the model revealed the known biochemical data was sufficient to create a situation where KRAS G13D cancers were relatively more sensitive highlights the difficulty of intuiting cellular behaviors on the basis of biochemical data without the aid of sophisticated mathematical models.

This study [90] further used the mathematical model to investigate the mechanism and predicted that the G13D-containing cancer was sensitive due to a greater reduction of wild-type RAS. That is, within a KRAS mutant cancer both the HRAS and NRAS genes are still typically wild-type and their gene products are wild-type. The model suggested that EGFR inhibition would better suppress HRAS-GTP and NRAS-GTP levels within the G13D cancers than in other RAS mutant cancers. Further analysis of the model suggested that the strength of interaction with NF1 was the critical variable; RAS mutants like KRAS G12D and KRAS G12V (the two most common KRAS mutants in colorectal cancer) bind NF1 strongly but nonproductively, and effectively competitively inhibit NF1 from acting on WT RAS and thereby shift the dynamic equilibrium to a higher level of WT RAS-GTP. In contrast, KRAS G13D is impaired at binding to NF1, so NF1 can reduce levels of WT RAS-GTP. In an EGFR-driven cancer, however, EGFR activation will result in increased WT RAS-GTP – and the targeting of EGFR will result in less WT RAS-GTP.

A separate study independently obtained very similar cell biological data using the same model systems, demonstrating that KRAS G13D cancer cells can reproducibly be observed to be sensitive to EGFR inhibitors [33]. Notably, the authors of that study also identified NF1 as a critical variable. However, they claim that NF1 can hydrolyze KRAS-G13D-GTP to KRAS-G13D-GDP conversion. Of note, we were unable to reproduce an effect at the scale of those authors in our own studies [32], and it appears that the authors of this other study may have used an antibody that binds HRAS, NRAS, and KRAS but then incorrectly attributed all differences in detected signal to KRAS [33]. Thus, it appears that wild-type RAS suppression is the mechanism by which KRAS G13D colorectal cancers benefit from EGFR inhibition. Both studies suggest that loss of NF1 activity will be a mechanism of resistance [33, 90]. Co-occurring NF1 mutations are common in KRAS G13D cell lines, but not in KRAS G13D patient samples [90], which suggests that NF1 loss of function is more likely to pose a challenge with acquired resistance. Nevertheless, these studies suggest that efforts to translate the KRAS G13D studies to patients may need to evaluate NF1 mutation status as a variable that may be able to identify the KRAS G13D patient population most likely to benefit from treatment with an EGFR inhibitor. If EGFR inhibition is clinically adopted for the treatment of KRAS G13D colorectal cancers, it will be interesting to determine whether NF1 loss of function is observed to be a mechanism of clinical resistance.

12 Summary

The field of RAS therapeutics has experienced an exciting rebirth, thanks to the development of KRAS G12C inhibitors. In addition to the promising potential of these agents to benefit KRAS G12C mutant lung cancer patients, these agents are motivating investigations into biophysically and biochemically exploitable features of other oncogenic RAS proteins. It seems reasonable to expect to see an increasing number of RAS-mutant specific therapies and RAS-mutant specific clinical trials. As these trials, which may include strategies that target the mutant RAS DNA, RNA, peptide, and protein, advance, it is important for clinicians to remember that different RAS proteins have distinct biochemical and biophysical properties that may provide the foundation for the distinct clinical responses.

References

[1] J. Canon, K. Rex, A. Y. Saiki, C. Mohr, K. Cooke, D. Bagal, K. Gaida, T. Holt, C. G. Knutson, N. Koppada, B. A. Lanman, J. Werner, A. S. Rapaport, T. San Miguel, R. Ortiz, T. Osgood, J. R. Sun, X. Zhu, J. D. McCarter, L. P. Volak, B. E. Houk, M. G. Fakih, B. H. O'Neil, T. J. Price, G. S. Falchook, J. Desai, J. Kuo, R. Govindan, D. S. Hong, W. Ouyang, H. Henary, T. Arvedson, V. J. Cee, J. R. Lipford, The clinical KRAS(G12C) inhibitor AMG 510 drives anti-tumour immunity. *Nature* **575**, 217–223 (2019); published online EpubNov (DOI: http://doi.org/10.1038/s41586-019-1694-1).

[2] C. Shih, R. A. Weinberg, Isolation of a transforming sequence from a human bladder carcinoma cell line. *Cell* **29**, 161–169 (1982); published online EpubMay (DOI: http://doi.org/10.1016/0092–8674 (82)90100–3).

[3] A. G. Stephen, D. Esposito, R. K. Bagni, F. McCormick, Dragging RAS back in the ring. *Cancer Cell* **25**, 272–281 (2014); published online EpubMar 17 (DOI: http://doi.org/10.1016/j.ccr.2014.02.017).

[4] S. Jones, X. Zhang, D. W. Parsons, J. C. Lin, R. J. Leary, P. Angenendt, P. Mankoo, H. Carter, H. Kamiyama, A. Jimeno, S. M. Hong, B. Fu, M. T. Lin, E. S. Calhoun, M. Kamiyama, K. Walter, T. Nikolskaya, Y. Nikolsky, J. Hartigan, D. R. Smith, M. Hidalgo, S. D. Leach, A. P. Klein, E. M. Jaffee, M. Goggins, A. Maitra, C. Iacobuzio-Donahue, J. R. Eshleman, S. E. Kern, R. H. Hruban, R. Karchin, N. Papadopoulos, G. Parmigiani, B. Vogelstein, V. E. Velculescu, K. W. Kinzler, Core signaling pathways in human pancreatic cancers revealed by global genomic analyses. *Science* **321**, 1801–1806 (2008); published online EpubSep 26 (DOI: http://doi.org/10.1126/science.1164368).

[5] Cancer Genome Atlas Research Network, Integrated genomic characterization of pancreatic ductal adenocarcinoma. *Cancer Cell* **32**, 185–203 e113 (2017); published online EpubAug 14 (DOI: http://doi.org/10.1016/j.ccell.2017.07.007).

[6] L. Ding, G. Getz, D. A. Wheeler, E. R. Mardis, M. D. McLellan, K. Cibulskis, C. Sougnez, H. Greulich, D. M. Muzny, M. B. Morgan, L. Fulton, R. S. Fulton, Q. Zhang, M. C. Wendl, M. S. Lawrence, D. E. Larson, K. Chen, D. J. Dooling, A. Sabo, A. C. Hawes, H. Shen, S. N. Jhangiani, L. R. Lewis, O. Hall, Y. Zhu, T. Mathew, Y. Ren, J. Yao, S. E. Scherer, K. Clerc, G. A. Metcalf, B. Ng, A. Milosavljevic, M. L. Gonzalez-Garay, J. R. Osborne, R. Meyer, X. Shi, Y. Tang, D. C. Koboldt, L. Lin, R. Abbott, T. L. Miner, C. Pohl, G. Fewell, C. Haipek, H. Schmidt, B. H. Dunford-Shore, A. Kraja, S. D. Crosby,

C. S. Sawyer, T. Vickery, S. Sander, J. Robinson, W. Winckler, J. Baldwin, L. R. Chirieac, A. Dutt, T. Fennell, M. Hanna, B. E. Johnson, R. C. Onofrio, R. K. Thomas, G. Tonon, B. A. Weir, X. Zhao, L. Ziaugra, M. C. Zody, T. Giordano, M. B. Orringer, J. A. Roth, M. R. Spitz, I. I. Wistuba, B. Ozenberger, P. J. Good, A. C. Chang, D. G. Beer, M. A. Watson, M. Ladanyi, S. Broderick, A. Yoshizawa, W. D. Travis, W. Pao, M. A. Province, G. M. Weinstock, H. E. Varmus, S. B. Gabriel, E. S. Lander, R. A. Gibbs, M. Meyerson, R. K. Wilson, Somatic mutations affect key pathways in lung adenocarcinoma. *Nature* **455**, 1069–1075 (2008); published online EpubOct 23 (DOI: http://doi.org/10.1038/nature07423).

[7] N. Cancer Genome Atlas, Comprehensive molecular characterization of human colon and rectal cancer. *Nature* **487**, 330–337 (2012); published online EpubJul 18 (DOI: http://doi.org/10.1038/nature11252).

[8] E. Hodis, I. R. Watson, G. V. Kryukov, S. T. Arold, M. Imielinski, J. P. Theurillat, E. Nickerson, D. Auclair, L. Li, C. Place, D. Dicara, A. H. Ramos, M. S. Lawrence, K. Cibulskis, A. Sivachenko, D. Voet, G. Saksena, N. Stransky, R. C. Onofrio, W. Winckler, K. Ardlie, N. Wagle, J. Wargo, K. Chong, D. L. Morton, K. Stemke-Hale, G. Chen, M. Noble, M. Meyerson, J. E. Ladbury, M. A. Davies, J. E. Gershenwald, S. N. Wagner, D. S. Hoon, D. Schadendorf, E. S. Lander, S. B. Gabriel, G. Getz, L. A. Garraway, L. Chin, A landscape of driver mutations in melanoma. *Cell* **150**, 251–263 (2012); published online EpubJul 20 (DOI: http://doi.org/10.1016/j.cell.2012.06.024).

[9] N. Cancer Genome Atlas, Comprehensive genomic characterization of head and neck squamous cell carcinomas. *Nature* **517**, 576–582 (2015); published online EpubJan 29 (DOI: http://doi.org/10.1038/nature 14129).

[10] G. Guo, X. Sun, C. Chen, S. Wu, P. Huang, Z. Li, M. Dean, Y. Huang, W. Jia, Q. Zhou, A. Tang, Z. Yang, X. Li, P. Song, X. Zhao, R. Ye, S. Zhang, Z. Lin, M. Qi, S. Wan, L. Xie, F. Fan, M. L. Nickerson, X. Zou, X. Hu, L. Xing, Z. Lv, H. Mei, S. Gao, C. Liang, Z. Gao, J. Lu, Y. Yu, C. Liu, L. Li, X. Fang, Z. Jiang, J. Yang, C. Li, X. Zhao, J. Chen, F. Zhang, Y. Lai, Z. Lin, F. Zhou, H. Chen, H. C. Chan, S. Tsang, D. Theodorescu, Y. Li, X. Zhang, J. Wang, H. Yang, Y. Gui, J. Wang, Z. Cai, Whole-genome and whole-exome sequencing of bladder cancer identifies frequent alterations in genes involved in sister chromatid cohesion and segregation. *Nat Genet* **45**, 1459–1463 (2013); published online EpubDec (DOI: http://doi.org/10.1038/ng.2798).

[11] D. Hanahan, R. A. Weinberg, The hallmarks of cancer. *Cell* **100**, 57–70 (2000); published online EpubJan 7 (DOI: http://doi.org/10.1016/s0092-8674(00)81683-9).

[12] D. Hanahan, R. A. Weinberg, Hallmarks of cancer: The next generation. *Cell* **144**, 646–674 (2011); published online EpubMar 4 (DOI: http://doi.org/10.1016/j.cell.2011.02.013).

[13] S. Mukhopadhyay, M. G. Vander Heiden, F. McCormick, The metabolic landscape of RAS-driven cancers from biology to therapy. *Nat Cancer* **2**, 271–283 (2021); published online EpubMar (DOI: http://doi.org/10.1038/s43018-021-00184-x).

[14] C. Commisso, S. M. Davidson, R. G. Soydaner-Azeloglu, S. J. Parker, J. J. Kamphorst, S. Hackett, E. Grabocka, M. Nofal, J. A. Drebin, C. B. Thompson, J. D. Rabinowitz, C. M. Metallo, M. G. Vander Heiden, D. Bar-Sagi, Macropinocytosis of protein is an amino acid supply route in Ras-transformed cells. *Nature* **497**, 633–637 (2013); published online EpubMay 30 (DOI: http://doi.org/10.1038/nature12138).

[15] E. M. Kerr, E. Gaude, F. K. Turrell, C. Frezza, C. P. Martins, Mutant *Kras* copy number defines metabolic reprogramming and therapeutic susceptibilities. *Nature* **531**, 110–113 (2016); published online EpubMar 3 (DOI: http://doi.org/10.1038/nature16967).

[16] A. Bonni, A. Brunet, A. E. West, S. R. Datta, M. A. Takasu, M. E. Greenberg, Cell survival promoted by the Ras-MAPK signaling pathway by transcription-dependent and -independent mechanisms. *Science* **286**, 1358–1362 (1999); published online EpubNov 12 (DOI: http://doi.org/10.1126/science.286.5443.1358).

[17] A. Kauffmann-Zeh, P. Rodriguez-Viciana, E. Ulrich, C. Gilbert, P. Coffer, J. Downward, G. Evan, Suppression of c-Myc-induced apoptosis by Ras signalling through PI(3)K and PKB. *Nature* **385**, 544–548 (1997); published online EpubFeb 6 (DOI: http://doi.org/10.1038/385544a0).

[18] M. V. Milburn, L. Tong, A. M. deVos, A. Brunger, Z. Yamaizumi, S. Nishimura, S. H. Kim, Molecular switch for signal transduction: Structural differences between active and inactive forms of protooncogenic RAS proteins. *Science* **247**, 939–945 (1990); published online EpubFeb 23 (DOI: http://doi.org/10.1126/science.2406906).

[19] H. Lavoie, M. Therrien, Regulation of RAF protein kinases in ERK signalling. *Nat Rev Mol Cell Biol* **16**, 281–298 (2015); published online EpubMay (DOI: http://doi.org/10.1038/nrm3979).

[20] J. C. Hunter, A. Manandhar, M. A. Carrasco, D. Gurbani, S. Gondi, K. D. Westover, Biochemical and structural analysis of common cancer-associated KRAS mutations. *Mol Cancer Res* **13**, 1325–1335 (2015); published online EpubSep (DOI: http://doi.org/10.1158/1541-7786.MCR-15-0203).

[21] M. R. Ahmadian, U. Hoffmann, R. S. Goody, A. Wittinghofer, Individual rate constants for the interaction of Ras proteins with GTPase-activating proteins determined by fluorescence spectroscopy. *Biochemistry* **36**, 4535–4541 (1997); published online EpubApr 15 (DOI: http://doi.org/10.1021/bi962556y).

[22] C. Lenzen, R. H. Cool, H. Prinz, J. Kuhlmann, A. Wittinghofer, Kinetic analysis by fluorescence of the interaction between Ras and the catalytic domain of the guanine nucleotide exchange factor Cdc25Mm. *Biochemistry* **37**, 7420–7430 (1998); published online EpubMay 19 (DOI: http://doi.org/10.1021/bi972621j).

[23] T. W. Traut, Physiological concentrations of purines and pyrimidines. *Mol Cell Biochem* **140**, 1–22 (1994); published online EpubNov 9 (DOI: http://doi.org/10.1007/BF00928361).

[24] X. Zhang, J. Gureasko, K. Shen, P. A. Cole, J. Kuriyan, An allosteric mechanism for activation of the kinase domain of epidermal growth factor receptor. *Cell* **125**, 1137–1149 (2006); published online EpubJun 16 (DOI: http://doi.org/10.1016/j.cell.2006.05.013).

[25] R. B. Jones, A. Gordus, J. A. Krall, G. MacBeath, A quantitative protein interaction network for the ErbB receptors using protein microarrays. *Nature* **439**, 168–174 (2006); published online EpubJan 12 (DOI: http://doi.org/10.1038/nature04177).

[26] K. S. Ravichandran, Signaling via Shc family adapter proteins. *Oncogene* **20**, 6322–6330 (2001); published online EpubOct 1 (DOI: http://doi.org/10.1038/sj.onc.1204776).

[27] A. M. Cheng, T. M. Saxton, R. Sakai, S. Kulkarni, G. Mbamalu, W. Vogel, C. G. Tortorice, R. D. Cardiff, J. C. Cross, W. J. Muller, T. Pawson, Mammalian Grb2 regulates multiple steps in embryonic development and malignant transformation. *Cell* **95**, 793–803 (1998); published online EpubDec 11 (DOI: http://doi.org/10.1016/s0092-8674(00)81702-x).

[28] G. Bollag, F. Adler, N. elMasry, P. C. McCabe, E. Conner, Jr., P. Thompson, F. McCormick, K. Shannon, Biochemical characterization of a novel KRAS insertion mutation from a human leukemia. *J Biol Chem* **271**, 32491–32494 (1996); published online EpubDec 20 (DOI: http://doi.org/10.1074/jbc.271.51.32491).

[29] S. Boykevisch, C. Zhao, H. Sondermann, P. Philippidou, S. Halegoua, J. Kuriyan, D. Bar-Sagi, Regulation of RAS signaling dynamics by Sos-mediated positive feedback. *Curr Biol* **16**, 2173–2179 (2006); published online EpubNov 7 (DOI: http://doi.org/10.1016/j.cub.2006.09.033).

[30] A. D. Cox, S. W. Fesik, A. C. Kimmelman, J. Luo, C. J. Der, Drugging the undruggable RAS: Mission possible? *Nat Rev Drug Discov* **13**, 828–851 (2014); published online EpubNov (DOI: http://doi.org/10.1038/nrd4389).

[31] M. J. Smith, B. G. Neel, M. Ikura, NMR-based functional profiling of RASopathies and oncogenic RAS mutations. *Proc Natl Acad Sci USA* **110**, 4574–4579 (2013); published online EpubMar 19 (DOI: http://doi.org/10.1073/pnas.1218173110).

[32] T. McFall, N. K. Schomburg, K. L. Rossman, E. C. Stites, Discernment between candidate mechanisms for KRAS G13D colorectal cancer sensitivity to EGFR inhibitors. *Cell Commun Signal* **18**, 179 (2020); published online EpubNov 5 (DOI: http://doi.org/10.1186/s12964-020-00645-3).

[33] D. Rabara, T. H. Tran, S. Dharmaiah, R. M. Stephens, F. McCormick, D. K. Simanshu, M. Holderfield, KRAS G13D sensitivity to neurofibromin-mediated GTP hydrolysis. *Proc Natl Acad Sci USA* **116**, 22122–22131 (2019); published online EpubOct 29 (DOI: http://doi.org/10.1073/pnas.1908353116).

[34] A. Singh, P. Greninger, D. Rhodes, L. Koopman, S. Violette, N. Bardeesy, J. Settleman, A gene expression signature associated with "K-Ras addiction" reveals regulators of EMT and tumor cell survival. *Cancer Cell* **15**, 489–500 (2009); published online EpubJun 2 (DOI: http://doi.org/10.1016/j.ccr.2009.03.022).

[35] A. Kapoor, W. Yao, H. Ying, S. Hua, A. Liewen, Q. Wang, Y. Zhong, C. J. Wu, A. Sadanandam, B. Hu, Q. Chang, G. C. Chu, R. Al-Khalil, S. Jiang, H. Xia, E. Fletcher-Sananikone, C. Lim, G. I. Horwitz, A. Viale, P. Pettazzoni, N. Sanchez, H. Wang, A. Protopopov, J. Zhang, T. Heffernan, R. L. Johnson, L. Chin, Y. A. Wang, G. Draetta, R. A. DePinho, Yap1 activation enables bypass of oncogenic Kras addiction in pancreatic cancer. *Cell* **158**, 185–197 (2014); published online EpubJul 3 (DOI: http://doi.org/10.1016/j.cell.2014.06.003).

[36] J. Luo, N. L. Solimini, S. J. Elledge, Principles of cancer therapy: Oncogene and non-oncogene addiction. *Cell* **136**, 823–837 (2009); published online EpubMar 6 (DOI: http://doi.org/10.1016/j.cell.2009.02.024).

[37] I. M. Ahearn, K. Haigis, D. Bar-Sagi, M. R. Philips, Regulating the regulator: Post-translational modification of RAS. *Nat Rev Mol Cell Biol* **13**, 39–51 (2011); published online EpubDec 22 (DOI: http://doi.org/10.1038/nrm3255).

[38] N. E. Kohl, C. A. Omer, M. W. Conner, N. J. Anthony, J. P. Davide, S. J. deSolms, E. A. Giuliani, R. P. Gomez, S. L. Graham, K. Hamilton,

et al., Inhibition of farnesyltransferase induces regression of mammary and salivary carcinomas in ras transgenic mice. *Nat Med* **1**, 792–797 (1995); published online EpubAug (DOI: http://doi.org/10.1038/nm 0895-792).

[39] D. B. Whyte, P. Kirschmeier, T. N. Hockenberry, I. Nunez-Oliva, L. James, J. J. Catino, W. R. Bishop, J. K. Pai, K- and N-Ras are geranylgeranylated in cells treated with farnesyl protein transferase inhibitors. *J Biol Chem* **272**, 14459–14464 (1997); published online EpubMay 30 (DOI: http://doi.org/10.1074/jbc.272.22.14459).

[40] C. A. Rowell, J. J. Kowalczyk, M. D. Lewis, A. M. Garcia, Direct demonstration of geranylgeranylation and farnesylation of Ki-Ras in vivo. *J Biol Chem* **272**, 14093–14097 (1997); published online EpubMay 30 (DOI: http://doi.org/10.1074/jbc.272.22.14093).

[41] H. W. Lee, J. K. Sa, A. Gualberto, C. Scholz, H. H. Sung, B. C. Jeong, H. Y. Choi, G. Y. Kwon, S. H. Park, A phase II trial of tipifarnib for patients with previously treated, metastatic urothelial carcinoma harboring HRAS mutations. *Clin Cancer Res* **26**, 5113–5119 (2020); published online EpubOct 1 (DOI: http://doi.org/10.1158/1078–0432.CCR-20–1246).

[42] A. L. Ho, I. Brana, R. Haddad, J. Bauman, K. Bible, S. Oosting, D. J. Wong, M. J. Ahn, V. Boni, C. Even, J. Fayette, M. J. Flor, K. Harrington, S. B. Kim, L. Licitra, I. Nixon, N. F. Saba, S. Hackenberg, P. Specenier, F. Worden, B. Balsara, M. Leoni, B. Martell, C. Scholz, A. Gualberto, Tipifarnib in head and neck squamous cell carcinoma with HRAS mutations. *J Clin Oncol* **39**, 1856–1864 (2021); published online EpubJun 10 (DOI: http://doi .org/10.1200/JCO.20.02903).

[43] G. Hatzivassiliou, K. Song, I. Yen, B. J. Brandhuber, D. J. Anderson, R. Alvarado, M. J. Ludlam, D. Stokoe, S. L. Gloor, G. Vigers, T. Morales, I. Aliagas, B. Liu, S. Sideris, K. P. Hoeflich, B. S. Jaiswal, S. Seshagiri, H. Koeppen, M. Belvin, L. S. Friedman, S. Malek, RAF inhibitors prime wild-type RAF to activate the MAPK pathway and enhance growth. *Nature* **464**, 431–435 (2010); published online EpubMar 18 (DOI: http:// doi.org/10.1038/nature08833).

[44] P. I. Poulikakos, C. Zhang, G. Bollag, K. M. Shokat, N. Rosen, RAF inhibitors transactivate RAF dimers and ERK signalling in cells with wild-type BRAF. *Nature* **464**, 427–430 (2010); published online EpubMar 18 (DOI: http://doi.org/10.1038/nature08902).

[45] F. Su, A. Viros, C. Milagre, K. Trunzer, G. Bollag, O. Spleiss, J. S. Reis-Filho, X. Kong, R. C. Koya, K. T. Flaherty, P. B. Chapman, M. J. Kim, R. Hayward, M. Martin, H. Yang, Q. Wang, H. Hilton, J. S. Hang, J. Noe, M. Lambros, F. Geyer, N. Dhomen, I. Niculescu-Duvaz, A. Zambon, D. Niculescu-Duvaz,

N. Preece, L. Robert, N. J. Otte, S. Mok, D. Kee, Y. Ma, C. Zhang, G. Habets, E. A. Burton, B. Wong, H. Nguyen, M. Kockx, L. Andries, B. Lestini, K. B. Nolop, R. J. Lee, A. K. Joe, J. L. Troy, R. Gonzalez, T. E. Hutson, I. Puzanov, B. Chmielowski, C. J. Springer, G. A. McArthur, J. A. Sosman, R. S. Lo, A. Ribas, R. Marais, RAS mutations in cutaneous squamous-cell carcinomas in patients treated with BRAF inhibitors. *N Engl J Med* **366**, 207–215 (2012); published online EpubJan 19 (DOI: http://doi.org/10.1056/NEJMoa1105358).

[46] C. Zhang, W. Spevak, Y. Zhang, E. A. Burton, Y. Ma, G. Habets, J. Zhang, J. Lin, T. Ewing, B. Matusow, G. Tsang, A. Marimuthu, H. Cho, G. Wu, W. Wang, D. Fong, H. Nguyen, S. Shi, P. Womack, M. Nespi, R. Shellooe, H. Carias, B. Powell, E. Light, L. Sanftner, J. Walters, J. Tsai, B. L. West, G. Visor, H. Rezaei, P. S. Lin, K. Nolop, P. N. Ibrahim, P. Hirth, G. Bollag, RAF inhibitors that evade paradoxical MAPK pathway activation. *Nature* **526**, 583–586 (2015); published online EpubOct 22 (DOI: http://doi.org/10.1038/nature14982).

[47] V. Chung, S. McDonough, P. A. Philip, D. Cardin, A. Wang-Gillam, L. Hui, M. A. Tejani, T. E. Seery, I. A. Dy, T. Al Baghdadi, A. E. Hendifar, L. A. Doyle, A. M. Lowy, K. A. Guthrie, C. D. Blanke, H. S. Hochster, Effect of selumetinib and MK-2206 vs oxaliplatin and fluorouracil in patients with metastatic pancreatic cancer after prior therapy: SWOG S1115 study randomized clinical trial. *JAMA Oncol* **3**, 516–522 (2017); published online EpubApr 1 (DOI: http://doi.org/10.1001/jamaoncol.2016.5383).

[48] K. Do, G. Speranza, R. Bishop, S. Khin, L. Rubinstein, R. J. Kinders, M. Datiles, M. Eugeni, M. H. Lam, L. A. Doyle, J. H. Doroshow, S. Kummar, Biomarker-driven phase 2 study of MK-2206 and selumetinib (AZD6244, ARRY-142886) in patients with colorectal cancer. *Invest New Drugs* **33**, 720–728 (2015); published online EpubJun (DOI: http://doi.org/10.1007/s10637-015-0212-z).

[49] E. Dombi, A. Baldwin, L. J. Marcus, M. J. Fisher, B. Weiss, A. Kim, P. Whitcomb, S. Martin, L. E. Aschbacher-Smith, T. A. Rizvi, J. Wu, R. Ershler, P. Wolters, J. Therrien, J. Glod, J. B. Belasco, E. Schorry, A. Brofferio, A. J. Starosta, A. Gillespie, A. L. Doyle, N. Ratner, B. C. Widemann, Activity of selumetinib in neurofibromatosis type 1-related plexiform neurofibromas. *N Engl J Med* **375**, 2550–2560 (2016); published online EpubDec 29 (DOI: http://doi.org/10.1056/NEJMoa1605943).

[50] J. K. Sicklick, S. Kato, R. Okamura, M. Schwaederle, M. E. Hahn, C. B. Williams, P. De, A. Krie, D. E. Piccioni, V. A. Miller, J. S. Ross, A. Benson, J. Webster, P. J. Stephens, J. J. Lee, P. T. Fanta, S. M. Lippman, B. Leyland-Jones, R. Kurzrock, Molecular profiling of cancer patients enables

personalized combination therapy: The I-PREDICT study. *Nat Med* **25**, 744–750 (2019); published online EpubMay (DOI: http://doi.org/10.1038/s41591-019–0407–5).

[51] S. Kato, K. H. Kim, H. J. Lim, A. Boichard, M. Nikanjam, E. Weihe, D. J. Kuo, R. N. Eskander, A. Goodman, N. Galanina, P. T. Fanta, R. B. Schwab, R. Shatsky, S. C. Plaxe, A. Sharabi, E. Stites, J. J. Adashek, R. Okamura, S. Lee, S. M. Lippman, J. K. Sicklick, R. Kurzrock, Real-world data from a molecular tumor board demonstrates improved outcomes with a precision N-of-One strategy. *Nat Commun* **11**, 4965 (2020); published online EpubOct 2 (DOI: http://doi.org/10.1038/s41467-020–18613–3).

[52] K. T. Flaherty, J. R. Infante, A. Daud, R. Gonzalez, R. F. Kefford, J. Sosman, O. Hamid, L. Schuchter, J. Cebon, N. Ibrahim, R. Kudchadkar, H. A. Burris, 3rd, G. Falchook, A. Algazi, K. Lewis, G. V. Long, I. Puzanov, P. Lebowitz, A. Singh, S. Little, P. Sun, A. Allred, D. Ouellet, K. B. Kim, K. Patel, J. Weber, Combined BRAF and MEK inhibition in melanoma with BRAF V600 mutations. *N Engl J Med* **367**, 1694–1703 (2012); published online EpubNov 1 (DOI: http://doi.org/10.1056/NEJMoa1210093).

[53] S. Kopetz, A. Grothey, R. Yaeger, E. Van Cutsem, J. Desai, T. Yoshino, H. Wasan, F. Ciardiello, F. Loupakis, Y. S. Hong, N. Steeghs, T. K. Guren, H. T. Arkenau, P. Garcia-Alfonso, P. Pfeiffer, S. Orlov, S. Lonardi, E. Elez, T. W. Kim, J. H. M. Schellens, C. Guo, A. Krishnan, J. Dekervel, V. Morris, A. Calvo Ferrandiz, L. S. Tarpgaard, M. Braun, A. Gollerkeri, C. Keir, K. Maharry, M. Pickard, J. Christy-Bittel, L. Anderson, V. Sandor, J. Tabernero, Encorafenib, binimetinib, and cetuximab in BRAF V600E-mutated colorectal cancer. *N Engl J Med* **381**, 1632–1643 (2019); published online EpubOct 24 (DOI: http://doi.org/10.1056/NEJMoa1908075).

[54] S. Kato, R. Okamura, J. K. Sicklick, G. A. Daniels, D. S. Hong, A. Goodman, E. Weihe, S. Lee, N. Khalid, R. Collier, M. Mareboina, P. Riviere, T. J. Whitchurch, P. T. Fanta, S. M. Lippman, R. Kurzrock, Prognostic implications of RAS alterations in diverse malignancies and impact of targeted therapies. *Int J Cancer* **146**, 3450–3460 (2020); published online EpubJun 15 (DOI: http://doi.org/10.1002/ijc.32813).

[55] S. Kato, T. McFall, K. Takahashi, K. Bamel, S. Ikeda, R. N. Eskander, S. Plaxe, B. Parker, E. Stites, R. Kurzrock, KRAS-mutated, estrogen receptor-positive low-grade serous ovarian cancer: Unraveling an exceptional response mystery. *Oncologist* **26**, e530–e536 (2021); published online EpubApr (DOI: http://doi.org/10.1002/onco.13702).

[56] S. Kato, J. J. Adashek, J. Shaya, R. Okamura, R. E. Jimenez, S. Lee, J. K. Sicklick, R. Kurzrock, Concomitant MEK and cyclin gene alterations: Implications for response to targeted therapeutics. *Clin Cancer Res* **27**,

2792–2797 (2021); published online EpubMay 15 (DOI: http://doi.org/10.1158/1078–0432.CCR-20–3761).

[57] C. S. Karapetis, S. Khambata-Ford, D. J. Jonker, C. J. O'Callaghan, D. Tu, N. C. Tebbutt, R. J. Simes, H. Chalchal, J. D. Shapiro, S. Robitaille, T. J. Price, L. Shepherd, H. J. Au, C. Langer, M. J. Moore, J. R. Zalcberg, K-ras mutations and benefit from cetuximab in advanced colorectal cancer. *N Engl J Med* **359**, 1757–1765 (2008); published online EpubOct 23 (DOI: http://doi.org/10.1056/NEJMoa0804385).

[58] W. Pao, T. Y. Wang, G. J. Riely, V. A. Miller, Q. Pan, M. Ladanyi, M. F. Zakowski, R. T. Heelan, M. G. Kris, H. E. Varmus, KRAS mutations and primary resistance of lung adenocarcinomas to gefitinib or erlotinib. *PLoS Med* **2**, e17 (2005); published online EpubJan (DOI: http://doi.org/10.1371/journal.pmed.0020017).

[59] M. J. Moore, D. Goldstein, J. Hamm, A. Figer, J. R. Hecht, S. Gallinger, H. J. Au, P. Murawa, D. Walde, R. A. Wolff, D. Campos, R. Lim, K. Ding, G. Clark, T. Voskoglou-Nomikos, M. Ptasynski, W. Parulekar, National Cancer Institute of Canada Clinical Trials Group, Erlotinib plus gemcitabine compared with gemcitabine alone in patients with advanced pancreatic cancer: A phase III trial of the National Cancer Institute of Canada Clinical Trials Group. *J Clin Oncol* **25**, 1960–1966 (2007); published online EpubMay 20 (DOI: http://doi.org/10.1200/JCO.2006.07.9525).

[60] W. De Roock, D. J. Jonker, F. Di Nicolantonio, A. Sartore-Bianchi, D. Tu, S. Siena, S. Lamba, S. Arena, M. Frattini, H. Piessevaux, E. Van Cutsem, C. J. O'Callaghan, S. Khambata-Ford, J. R. Zalcberg, J. Simes, C. S. Karapetis, A. Bardelli, S. Tejpar, Association of KRAS p.G13D mutation with outcome in patients with chemotherapy-refractory metastatic colorectal cancer treated with cetuximab. *Jama* **304**, 1812–1820 (2010); published online EpubOct 27 (DOI: http://doi.org/10.1001/jama.2010.1535).

[61] S. Tejpar, I. Celik, M. Schlichting, U. Sartorius, C. Bokemeyer, E. Van Cutsem, Association of KRAS G13D tumor mutations with outcome in patients with metastatic colorectal cancer treated with first-line chemotherapy with or without cetuximab. *J Clin Oncol* **30**, 3570–3577 (2012); published online EpubOct 10 (DOI: http://doi.org/10.1200/JCO.2012.42.2592).

[62] R. C. Hillig, B. Sautier, J. Schroeder, D. Moosmayer, A. Hilpmann, C. M. Stegmann, N. D. Werbeck, H. Briem, U. Boemer, J. Weiske, V. Badock, J. Mastouri, K. Petersen, G. Siemeister, J. D. Kahmann, D. Wegener, N. Bohnke, K. Eis, K. Graham, L. Wortmann, F. von Nussbaum, B. Bader, Discovery of potent SOS1 inhibitors that block

RAS activation via disruption of the RAS-SOS1 interaction. *Proc Natl Acad Sci USA* **116**, 2551–2560 (2019); published online EpubFeb 12 (DOI: http://doi.org/10.1073/pnas.1812963116).

[63] M. C. Burns, Q. Sun, R. N. Daniels, D. Camper, J. P. Kennedy, J. Phan, E. T. Olejniczak, T. Lee, A. G. Waterson, O. W. Rossanese, S. W. Fesik, Approach for targeting Ras with small molecules that activate SOS-mediated nucleotide exchange. *Proc Natl Acad Sci USA* **111**, 3401–3406 (2014); published online EpubMar 4 (DOI: http://doi.org/10 .1073/pnas.1315798111).

[64] T. Maurer, L. S. Garrenton, A. Oh, K. Pitts, D. J. Anderson, N. J. Skelton, B. P. Fauber, B. Pan, S. Malek, D. Stokoe, M. J. Ludlam, K. K. Bowman, J. Wu, A. M. Giannetti, M. A. Starovasnik, I. Mellman, P. K. Jackson, J. Rudolph, W. Wang, G. Fang, Small-molecule ligands bind to a distinct pocket in Ras and inhibit SOS-mediated nucleotide exchange activity. *Proc Natl Acad Sci USA* **109**, 5299–5304 (2012); published online EpubApr 3 (DOI: http://doi.org/10.1073/pnas.1116510109).

[65] D. L. Kerr, F. Haderk, T. G. Bivona, Allosteric SHP2 inhibitors in cancer: Targeting the intersection of RAS, resistance, and the immune microenvironment. *Curr Opin Chem Biol* **62**, 1–12 (2021); published online EpubJan 6 (DOI: http://doi.org/10.1016/j.cbpa.2020.11.007).

[66] E. C. Stites, P. C. Trampont, Z. Ma, K. S. Ravichandran, Network analysis of oncogenic Ras activation in cancer. *Science* **318**, 463–467 (2007); published online EpubOct 19 (DOI: http://doi.org/10.1126/science .1144642).

[67] S. Kato, R. Porter, R. Okamura, S. Lee, O. Zelichov, G. Tarcic, M. Vidne, R. Kurzrock, Functional measurement of mitogen-activated protein kinase pathway activation predicts responsiveness of RAS-mutant cancers to MEK inhibitors. *Eur J Cancer* **149**, 184–192 (2021); published online EpubMay (DOI: http://doi.org/10.1016/j.ejca.2021.01.055).

[68] N. Cancer Genome Atlas Research, Comprehensive molecular profiling of lung adenocarcinoma. *Nature* **511**, 543–550 (2014); published online EpubJul 31 (DOI: http://doi.org/10.1038/nature13385).

[69] J. M. Ostrem, U. Peters, M. L. Sos, J. A. Wells, K. M. Shokat, K- Ras (G12C) inhibitors allosterically control GTP affinity and effector interactions. *Nature* **503**, 548–551 (2013); published online EpubNov 28 (DOI: http://doi.org/10.1038/nature12796).

[70] M. P. Patricelli, M. R. Janes, L. S. Li, R. Hansen, U. Peters, L. V. Kessler, Y. Chen, J. M. Kucharski, J. Feng, T. Ely, J. H. Chen, S. J. Firdaus, A. Babbar, P. Ren, Y. Liu, Selective inhibition of oncogenic KRAS output with small molecules targeting the inactive state. *Cancer Discov* **6**,

316–329 (2016); published online EpubMar (DOI: http://doi.org/10.1158/2159-8290.CD-15-1105).

[71] J. Hallin, L. D. Engstrom, L. Hargis, A. Calinisan, R. Aranda, D. M. Briere, N. Sudhakar, V. Bowcut, B. R. Baer, J. A. Ballard, M. R. Burkard, J. B. Fell, J. P. Fischer, G. P. Vigers, Y. Xue, S. Gatto, J. Fernandez-Banet, A. Pavlicek, K. Velastagui, R. C. Chao, J. Barton, M. Pierobon, E. Baldelli, E. F. Patricoin, 3rd, D. P. Cassidy, M. A. Marx, I. I. Rybkin, M. L. Johnson, S. I. Ou, P. Lito, K. P. Papadopoulos, P. A. Janne, P. Olson, J. G. Christensen, The KRAS(G12C) inhibitor MRTX849 provides insight toward therapeutic susceptibility of KRAS-mutant cancers in mouse models and patients. *Cancer Discov* **10**, 54–71 (2020); published online EpubJan (DOI: http://doi.org/10.1158/2159-8290.CD-19-1167).

[72] D. S. Hong, M. G. Fakih, J. H. Strickler, J. Desai, G. A. Durm, G. I. Shapiro, G. S. Falchook, T. J. Price, A. Sacher, C. S. Denlinger, Y. J. Bang, G. K. Dy, J. C. Krauss, Y. Kuboki, J. C. Kuo, A. L. Coveler, K. Park, T. W. Kim, F. Barlesi, P. N. Munster, S. S. Ramalingam, T. F. Burns, F. Meric-Bernstam, H. Henary, J. Ngang, G. Ngarmchamnanrith, J. Kim, B. E. Houk, J. Canon, J. R. Lipford, G. Friberg, P. Lito, R. Govindan, B. T. Li, KRAS(G12C) inhibition with sotorasib in advanced solid tumors. *N Engl J Med* **383**, 1207–1217 (2020); published online EpubSep 24 (DOI: http://doi.org/10.1056/NEJMoa1917239).

[73] P. Lito, M. Solomon, L. S. Li, R. Hansen, N. Rosen, Allele-specific inhibitors inactivate mutant KRAS G12C by a trapping mechanism. *Science* **351**, 604–608 (2016); published online EpubFeb 5 (DOI: http://doi.org/10.1126/science.aad6204).

[74] S. Misale, J. P. Fatherree, E. Cortez, C. Li, S. Bilton, D. Timonina, D. T. Myers, D. Lee, M. Gomez-Caraballo, M. Greenberg, V. Nangia, P. Greninger, R. K. Egan, J. McClanaghan, G. T. Stein, E. Murchie, P. P. Zarrinkar, M. R. Janes, L. S. Li, Y. Liu, A. N. Hata, C. H. Benes, KRAS G12C NSCLC models are sensitive to direct targeting of KRAS in combination with PI3K inhibition. *Clin Cancer Res* **25**, 796–807 (2019); published online EpubJan 15 (DOI: http://doi.org/10.1158/1078-0432.CCR-18-0368).

[75] K. Lou, V. Steri, A. Y. Ge, Y. C. Hwang, C. H. Yogodzinski, A. R. Shkedi, A. L. M. Choi, D. C. Mitchell, D. L. Swaney, B. Hann, J. D. Gordan, K. M. Shokat, L. A. Gilbert, KRAS(G12C) inhibition produces a driver-limited state revealing collateral dependencies. *Sci Signal* **12** (2019); published online EpubMay 28 (DOI: http://doi.org/10.1126/scisignal.aaw9450).

[76] M. B. Ryan, F. Fece de la Cruz, S. Phat, D. T. Myers, E. Wong, H. A. Shahzade, C. B. Hong, R. B. Corcoran, Vertical pathway inhibition overcomes adaptive feedback resistance to KRASG12C inhibition. *Clin Cancer Res* **26**, 1633–1643 (2019); published online EpubNov 27 (DOI: http://doi.org/10.1158/1078–0432.CCR-19–3523).

[77] M. P. Zafra, M. J. Parsons, J. Kim, D. Alonso-Curbelo, S. Goswami, E. M. Schatoff, T. Han, A. Katti, M. T. Calvo Fernandez, J. E. Wilkinson, E. Piskounova, L. E. Dow, An in vivo KRAS allelic series reveals distinct phenotypes of common oncogenic variants. *Cancer Discov* (2020); published online EpubAug 12 (DOI: http://doi.org/10.1158/2159–8290.CD-20–0442).

[78] V. Amodio, R. Yaeger, P. Arcella, C. Cancelliere, S. Lamba, A. Lorenzato, S. Arena, M. Montone, B. Mussolin, Y. Bian, A. Whaley, M. Pinnelli, Y. R. Murciano-Goroff, E. Vakiani, N. Valeri, W. L. Liao, A. Bhalkikar, S. Thyparambil, H. Y. Zhao, E. de Stanchina, S. Marsoni, S. Siena, A. Bertotti, L. Trusolino, B. T. Li, N. Rosen, F. Di Nicolantonio, A. Bardelli, S. Misale, EGFR blockade reverts resistance to KRAS (G12C) inhibition in colorectal cancer. *Cancer Discov* **10**, 1129–1139 (2020); published online EpubAug (DOI: http://doi.org/10.1158/2159–8290.CD-20–0187).

[79] G. A. Hobbs, A. Wittinghofer, C. J. Der, Selective targeting of the KRAS G12C mutant: Kicking KRAS when it's down. *Cancer Cell* **29**, 251–253 (2016); published online EpubMar 14 (DOI: http://doi.org/10.1016/j.ccell.2016.02.015).

[80] R. B. Corcoran, H. Ebi, A. B. Turke, E. M. Coffee, M. Nishino, A. P. Cogdill, R. D. Brown, P. Della Pelle, D. Dias-Santagata, K. E. Hung, K. T. Flaherty, A. Piris, J. A. Wargo, J. Settleman, M. Mino-Kenudson, J. A. Engelman, EGFR-mediated re-activation of MAPK signaling contributes to insensitivity of BRAF mutant colorectal cancers to RAF inhibition with vemurafenib. *Cancer Discov* **2**, 227–235 (2012); published online EpubMar (DOI: http://doi.org/10.1158/2159–8290.CD-11–0341).

[81] A. Prahallad, C. Sun, S. Huang, F. Di Nicolantonio, R. Salazar, D. Zecchin, R. L. Beijersbergen, A. Bardelli, R. Bernards, Unresponsiveness of colon cancer to BRAF(V600E) inhibition through feedback activation of EGFR. *Nature* **483**, 100–103 (2012); published online EpubMar 1 (DOI: http://doi.org/10.1038/nature10868).

[82] N. S. Akhave, A. B. Biter, D. S. Hong, Mechanisms of resistance to KRAS (G12C)-targeted therapy. *Cancer Discov* **11**, 1345–1352 (2021); published online EpubJun (DOI: http://doi.org/10.1158/2159–8290.CD-20–1616).

[83] N. Tanaka, J. J. Lin, C. Li, M. B. Ryan, J. Zhang, L. A. Kiedrowski, A. G. Michel, M. U. Syed, K. A. Fella, M. Sakhi, I. Baiev, D. Juric, J. F. Gainor, S. J. Klempner, J. K. Lennerz, G. Siravegna, L. Bar-Peled, A. N. Hata, R. S. Heist, R. B. Corcoran, Clinical acquired resistance to KRASG12C inhibition through a novel KRAS switch-II pocket mutation and polyclonal alterations converging on RAS-MAPK reactivation. *Cancer Discov* **11**, 1913–1922 (2021); published online EpubApr 6 (DOI: http://doi.org/10.1158/2159–8290.CD-21–0365).

[84] Y. Zhang, J. A. Ma, H. X. Zhang, Y. N. Jiang, W. H. Luo, Cancer vaccines: Targeting KRAS-driven cancers. *Expert Rev Vaccines* **19**, 163–173 (2020); published online EpubFeb (DOI: http://doi.org/10.1080/14760584.2020.1733420).

[85] G. A. Hobbs, N. M. Baker, A. M. Miermont, R. D. Thurman, M. Pierobon, T. H. Tran, A. O. Anderson, A. M. Waters, J. N. Diehl, B. Papke, R. G. Hodge, J. E. Klomp, C. M. Goodwin, J. M. DeLiberty, J. Wang, R. W. S. Ng, P. Gautam, K. L. Bryant, D. Esposito, S. L. Campbell, E. F. Petricoin, D. K. Simanshu, A. J. Aguirre, B. M. Wolpin, K. Wennerberg, U. Rudloff, A. D. Cox, C. J. Der, Atypical KRAS (G12R) mutant is impaired in PI3K signaling and macropinocytosis in pancreatic cancer. *Cancer Discov* **10**, 104–123 (2020); published online EpubJan (DOI: http://doi.org/10.1158/2159–8290.CD-19–1006).

[86] NCCN, *NCCN Guidelines Version 2.2017 Colon Cancer* (2017).

[87] M. P. Morelli, S. Kopetz, Hurdles and complexities of codon 13 KRAS mutations. *J Clin Oncol* **30**, 3565–3567 (2012); published online EpubOct 10 (DOI: http://doi.org/10.1200/JCO.2012.43.6535).

[88] M. Peeters, J. Y. Douillard, E. Van Cutsem, S. Siena, K. Zhang, R. Williams, J. Wiezorek, Mutant KRAS codon 12 and 13 alleles in patients with metastatic colorectal cancer: Assessment as prognostic and predictive biomarkers of response to panitumumab. *J Clin Oncol* **31**, 759–765 (2013); published online EpubFeb 20 (DOI: http://doi.org/10.1200/JCO.2012.45.1492).

[89] L. Gremer, B. Gilsbach, M. R. Ahmadian, A. Wittinghofer, Fluoride complexes of oncogenic Ras mutants to study the Ras-RasGap interaction. *Biol Chem* **389**, 1163–1171 (2008); published online EpubSep (DOI: http://doi.org/10.1515/BC.2008.132).

[90] T. McFall, J. K. Diedrich, M. Mengistu, S. L. Littlechild, K. V. Paskvan, L. Sisk-Hackworth, J. J. Moresco, A. S. Shaw, E. C. Stites, A systems mechanism for KRAS mutant allele-specific responses to targeted therapy. *Sci Signal* **12** (2019); published online EpubSep 24 (DOI: http://doi.org/10.1126/scisignal.aaw8288).

[91] M. Nakamura, T. Aoyama, K. Ishibashi, A. Tsuji, Y. Takinishi, Y. Shindo, J. Sakamoto, K. Oba, H. Mishima, Randomized phase II study of cetuximab versus irinotecan and cetuximab in patients with chemo-refractory KRAS codon G13D metastatic colorectal cancer (G13D-study). *Cancer Chemother Pharmacol* **79**, 29–36 (2017); published online EpubJan (DOI: http://doi.org/10.1007/s00280-016-3203-7).

[92] E. Segelov, S. Thavaneswaran, P. M. Waring, J. Desai, K. P. Robledo, V. J. Gebski, E. Elez, L. M. Nott, C. S. Karapetis, S. Lunke, L. A. Chantrill, N. Pavlakis, M. Khasraw, C. Underhill, F. Ciardiello, M. Jefford, H. Wasan, A. Haydon, T. J. Price, G. van Hazel, K. Wilson, J. Simes, J. D. Shapiro, Response to cetuximab with or without irinotecan in patients with refractory metastatic colorectal cancer harboring the KRAS G13D mutation: Australasian gastro-intestinal trials group ICECREAM study. *J Clin Oncol* **34**, 2258–2264 (2016); published online EpubJul 1 (DOI: http://doi.org/10.1200/JCO.2015.65.6843).

Acknowledgments

Support for this work was provided by the American Lung Association Lung Cancer Discovery Award, DOD W81XWH2010538, and by NIH DP2 AT011327.

Molecular Oncology

Edward P. Gelmann

University of Arizona

Dr. Edward P. Gelmann is John Norton Professor of Prostate Cancer Research at the University of Arizona and the University of Arizona Cancer Center. Dr. Gelmann previously headed Divisions of Hematology/Oncology at both Georgetown University and Columbia University. He has been the recipient of NIH, DOD and NIEHS grants for his research that has spanned cancer basic, clinical, and population sciences. Dr. Gelmann's research currently focuses on the early stages of prostate carcinogenesis and the development of novel therapeutics for prostate cancer. He continues to be involved in clinical care and clinical research of genitourinary malignancies. He has an active clinical practice and directs GU clinical research at the Cancer Center. Dr. Gelmann has published extensively and is senior editor of the book *Molecular Oncology: Causes of Cancer and Targets for Treatment* (Cambridge University Press, 2013).

About the Series

Therapeutics in clinical oncology are based increasingly on molecular drivers and hallmarks of cancers. *Elements in Molecular Oncology* provides a timely overview of topics in oncology for researchers and clinicians. By focusing on cancer sites or pathways, this series presents information on the latest findings on cancer causation and treatment.

Cambridge Elements ≡

Molecular Oncology

Elements in the Series

Personalized Drug Screening for Functional Tumor Profiling
Victoria El-Khoury, Tatiana Michel, Hichul Kim, and Yong-Jun Kwon

Therapeutic Targeting of RAS Mutant Cancers
Edward C. Stites, Kendra Paskvan, and Shumei Kato